Mysterious Healing Secrets from Around the World

CONTRIBUTING WRITER:

Jeffrey Laign

Publications International, Ltd.

Jeffrey Laign is a writer and editor with a special involvement in herbs and natural healing. An author of many magazine articles and books, including *The Complete Book of Herbs,* he has also been managing editor for Health Communications, Inc.

DISCLAIMER:
    Neither Publications International, Ltd., nor the author or publisher takes responsibility for any possible consequences from any treatment, procedure, exercise, dietary modification, action, or application of medication or preparation by any person reading or following the information in this book. This publication does not attempt to replace your physician or other health care provider. Before undertaking any course of treatment or dietary modification, the publisher and author advise you to check with your doctor or other health care provider.

CONTENTS

A World of Medical Mysteries

A Kansas woman asks fellow church members to pray for her before she has cancer surgery. A doctor in California inserts hair-thin needles in a man suffering from high blood pressure. A grandmother in Pennsylvania promises to cure a painful skin condition by waving a red string and chanting.

For those of us whose health depends on the scientific miracles of Western medicine, such remedies may seem silly, strange, and even barbaric. But for most people living in the world, medicine is a mix of mysterious healing secrets. Potions, powders, and poultices, in fact, are the first line of treatment for more than 80 percent of the world's population.

Even more amazing is that many seemingly bizarre medical practices actually work, although science has yet to figure out how. From country to country, culture to culture, healing rituals are as varied as the illnesses they treat. But all mysterious healing techniques seem to have one common thread—the belief that mind and body are strongly connected. It's only been recently that Western doctors have begun to appreciate what tribal healers have said for centuries: If you believe something will heal you, it may indeed help you to get well.

The link between mind and body appears to be a powerful one, a link that is not easily broken or ignored.

But it is a link that is shrouded in mystery. How, for example, could a man on his deathbed get up and walk again after asking a higher power for help? Sounds strange, but it's happened in every corner of the world.

The Power of Faith

A survey published in 1986 revealed that one of every seven people polled believed that at some point he or she had been healed by God. Such miraculous cures were for all types of illnesses—everything from viral conditions to debilitating back pain and cancer.

No one can say how prayer heals. But that doesn't stop people from praying. A 1991 study found that 96 percent of patients facing heart surgery said they prayed to be healed; 73 percent of hospitalized patients said the same thing in a study two years later.

Religion seeks to bring humans closer to the mysteries of the universe. And it appears that strong religious beliefs can protect or heal us from illness. In 1982, researchers found that Mormon men who considered themselves very religious were less likely to get cancer than their less-religious peers. What's more, if they did get cancer, those in the religious group recovered faster.

Similar results were published in a 1990 edition of the *American Journal of Psychiatry*, which reported that religious people recovered faster from illnesses and were less depressed than respondents who did not rate religion highly in their lives.

But here's the truly strange part. You don't have to go to church or even believe in God to reap the same mind-body rewards enjoyed by the devout. Many studies have concluded that people have been healed by simply slowing down and relaxing or by "willing" themselves to be well.

Meditation, for example, has been used to improve the symptoms of myriad illnesses, including high blood pressure, pain, and anxiety disorders. Think of meditation as a mental exercise aimed at training the mind to let go and become free. When people meditate on a regular basis, they often find that they become more resilient to life's ups and downs and are able to ward off or get rid of any number of ailments.

Guided imagery, a form of meditation in which people relax while listening to descriptions of positive images—from a tape or a therapist—also has been credited with producing miraculous cures. Doctors have been astounded by cancer patients who rid themselves of tumors by "willing" cancer cells to shrink and disappear. How could such a thing be possible? It's a mystery to science.

Smell and Touch

At the other end of the spectrum, nurturing the body can heal the mind and the illnesses that may originate there. Touch therapy is one of the oldest forms of healing in the world, as old as humans' natural instinct to rub the spot that hurts. In the Pyrenees Mountains that separate France and Spain, anthropologists have discovered depictions of people using touch to heal in cave paintings that date to 15,000 B.C.

Today thousands of people around the world swear by the healing miracles of touch therapies, from Swedish massage to Japanese shiatsu.

Aromatherapy is another mysterious mind-body medicine that has gained tremendous popularity in recent years. How can smelling something cure you of an illness? Nobody knows exactly. But people have been practicing this alternative medical technique for thousands of years—and they often get results.

Aromatherapy probably arose from the accidental discovery that some firewoods, such as cypress and cedar, fill the air with scents that make people feel better. The word perfume, in fact, is derived from the Latin *per fumum*, which means "through smoke." Thus, early aromatherapists healed patients by burning incense made from fragrant woods, leaves, needles, and gums.

Modern aromatherapists use essential oils from herbs and other plants to treat a number of ailments and to promote physical and emotional well-being. Often these scents are heavenly. But, strangely enough, healers once used noxious odors to treat people, too.

Equally perplexing is the use of rocks, crystals, amulets, and other objects to achieve healing. In India, practitioners of the ancient healing system of Ayurveda still make potions by pulverizing minerals, metals, and gemstones and mixing the powder with herbs.

Mind-body therapies spring from traditions as old as humankind. Shamanism is perhaps the first kind of medicine ever practiced. But it is more than just medicine. Shamanism is a way to see and make sense of the world, and many cultures in all parts of the globe still hold a variety of shamanic beliefs.

Shamans use power objects, such as drums and rattles, to achieve an altered state of consciousness and enter the spirit world. Here, they believe, lies the root of all sickness and disease. A shaman heals a patient only by entering that world and intervening with the spirits.

Asian Mysteries

Historians once considered Siberia the birthplace of shamanism. In Siberia, the shaman seemed to have been more central to the life of his people than anywhere else in the world. In fact, the word shaman derives from a Siberian language and describes a man or woman who has learned to master the mysterious forces of life and death.

Shamanism was the common heritage of the Stone Age way of life across Europe, Asia, and the Americas. There are powerful traces of traditional shamanism, for example, in the religions of Buddhism and Lamaism.

Buddhist healing philosophy figures heavily in the mysterious healing practices of Tibet. Because Buddhist medicine views all knowledge of healing as the gift of a compassionate Buddha to a suffering world, Tibetan physicians consider compassion to be the heart of their work and a prerequisite for effective healing.

Tibetan Buddhist healers see the world as one among many, and the present as a mere moment in a cycle of creation and destruction that extends through the vast reaches of time.

Such concepts are echoed in China, which enjoys one of the richest traditions of healing arts in the world. Ancient Chinese physicians were acquainted with more than 5,000 healing substances, including herbs, minerals, and animal parts. Today, Chinese doctors still prescribe remedies using many of those ingredients. In fact, numerous aspects of Chinese medicine bear more than a passing resemblance to the healing techniques of the people who lived in China more than 2,000 years ago.

Central to Chinese healing is the concept of *yin* and *yang*. The *yin-yang* school explains the world in terms of paired opposites. *Yin* is said to represent "female," or receptive energy; *yang*, "male," or penetrating energy. In Chinese medicine, the body's organs and systems can be organized in terms of *yin* and *yang*.

Also essential to understanding Chinese medicine is *qi* (chee), the mysterious energy that Chinese physicians believe animates all matter. This energy is thought to flow through the body along a system of channels. When the flow of *qi* is blocked, disease arises.

Chinese physicians attempt to correct a *qi* imbalance with acupuncture. They stimulate and manipulate the flow of *qi* by inserting hair-thin needles in specific points on the body that correspond to various body organs. Sometimes acupuncture is combined with moxibustion, in which powdered leaves of the herb mugwort (*Artemesia vulgaris*) are placed on or near the energy point and burned. No needles are used with a similar therapy, acupressure. Instead, energy points are pressed or massaged to achieve a therapeutic effect.

The principles of Chinese medicine were exported throughout Asia, from Singapore to Korea and Japan. With some slight variations, most of the theories underlying traditional Japanese medicine are identical to those of traditional Chinese medicine. *Yin* and *yang* and *ki*, the Japanese version of the Chinese *qi*, came to be the important organizing principles in Japan, just as they did in China. The Japanese also combined *amma*, a type of massage, with acupuncture concepts to create a system of healing massage known as *shiatsu*.

India is another Asian country that developed a coherent medical system whose tenets remain in practice today. That 5,000-year-old system, called Ayurveda, is still practiced throughout the Indian subcontinent and is enjoying a burgeoning popularity in the West.

In Sanskrit, the language of ancient India, Ayurveda means the "science of longevity" or "science of life." Ayurveda seeks to restore harmony and balance to the body, mind, and spirit through a system of diet, herbal medicine, massage, purification, and lifestyle discipline.

Many practitioners of Ayurveda also recommend yoga. Yoga uses a psychological and physiological system of exercise to gain control of and exercise both body and mind, thereby freeing the spirit. Although yoga is not a healing system like Ayurveda or traditional Chinese medicine, it strongly encourages and promotes the good health of its practitioners.

As in Asia, many American healing traditions are rooted in mysterious shamanic concepts. That's not surprising when you consider that the people who first lived in the Western hemisphere traveled here millennia ago across a once-existent land bridge between Alaska and Siberia.

Native American Traditions

Native Americans were able to preserve their healing traditions from the time of the first migrations out of Asia—perhaps 40,000 years ago—until Europeans displaced their cultures in the 16th century.

Among Indians in North and South America, shamans were central to the religious life and physical and mental health of the people in their communities. Although traditions varied widely among tribes, most North American Indians relied on healing ceremonies and other forms of spiritual medicine.

North American Indians also had a vast knowledge of the healing power of plants. In fact, they were familiar with more than 18,000 medicinal uses of plants, according to a 1986 University of Michigan study.

Herbal medicine was also practiced by the Aztec and Maya Indians of Mexico and Central America and by the Incas of Peru. Early Spanish chroniclers noted that the Aztecs used more than 500 healing plants.

To an Aztec, the world was full of spirits. Human beings were said to be filled with *tonalli,* an animating energy similar to the Chinese *qi* that manifested in body heat and blood. To treat an illness, an Aztec physician might go on a spirit quest to recover a patient's lost *tonalli* and then force out a disease-provoking spirit by sucking it from the patient by mouth or through a tube.

Farther south, the Maya, who thrived from about A.D. 200 to A.D. 800, practiced similar rituals to manipulate an energy similar in concept to *tonalli*. Mayas also practiced blood-letting, like their European counterparts, and prescribed purgative enemas.

In the vast Inca empire, stretching along the west coast of South America, healers used hundreds of medicinal plants and performed a crude sort of brain surgery by drilling small holes in a patient's head to relieve pressure or allow disease to escape.

Baffling Beliefs

Although many mysterious medical practices have been lost to the ages, others survive in full force. Herbalism, for example, has been undergoing a renaissance in the United States for the last several years, with annual sales of herbal products in the millions of dollars. Herbal medicine is popular in Asia, India, and Europe as well.

Modern conventional medicine owes much to its herbal past. Drug companies still use the natural plant world as a source of many pharmaceutical medicines. Seventy-seven percent of the 150 most commonly prescribed drugs today are of plant origin.

Also growing in popularity is an unusual therapy called homeopathy. The word derives from the Greek words *homeo* (similar) and *pathos* (suffering from disease). Developed in 1796 by German chemist and physician Samuel Hahnemann, homeopathy is based on the principle of similars—that is, that an infinitesimal dose of a substance can heal the symptoms caused by a larger amount of the same substance. Some home-opathic medicines are so diluted that the main ingredient is virtually nonexistent. And yet thousands of people testify that homeopathy has saved their lives.

Equally baffling but popular is chiropractic. Chiropractic—from the Greek for "done by hand"—was born in 1895 after Daniel Palmer, an Iowa grocer, reputedly restored a local janitor's hearing by manipulating his spine. Palmer had come up with the notion that nearly all diseases result from nerves pinched by misaligned vertebrae. You have 24 of these moveable bones protecting your spinal cord, and between each are nerves extending to all parts of your body. The spine, Palmer reasoned, was a pathway to the brain. Thus, he theorized, a spinal malformity could cause all sorts of ills, while realignment could heal.

Melting Pot Medicine

The United States, of course, is a land of immigrants, and many of the ethnic groups that have settled here brought with them mysterious healing secrets. Among the strangest are those practiced by the Amish, German Protestants who came to America in search of religious freedom. Although Amish communities are spread over 20 states, large groups live in Pennsylvania.

The Amish have always been a mystery to most Americans. That's because they shun the modern world and its conveniences, including automobiles, electricity, telephones, TVs, and computers. Even stranger are their medical beliefs. Many Amish view disease as an act of

God. Although some Amish take advantage of modern medicine when necessary, others stick to the old traditions, including Powwow medicine, whose practitioners use spells, chants, and hexes to rid the body of disease.

Some of the oldest influences in African-American folk medicine come from the combination of West African religions and the Roman Catholicism of white slave masters, especially in the Caribbean and Latin America. These influences led to the development of distinctive religions with strong African roots, such as voodoo, which also was used to heal. Africans brought to this country as slaves brought voodoo with them, along with strange healing therapies that were appreciated even by some white colonists. For example, Cotton Mather, the famous Puritan minister in Massachusetts, wrote that he learned how to treat smallpox from an enslaved African. African-American folk medicine has a rich and varied herbal tradition, especially in the rural South. But perhaps the most dominant form of healing among African-Americans is prayer—prayer by the patient, family, pastor, and congregation.

Faith also plays a large role in Asian-American healing mysteries. The Hmong people, who came here after 1976 from the mountains of Laos and Vietnam, believe that spirits in nature may cause illness if they have been angered. The Hmongs also believe that people have more than one soul. Losing a soul, or several, they believe, is one of the main causes of illness.

Visit a *botanica* in Miami or New York and you'll find scores of herbal remedies to treat *ataques de nervios,* or nervous attacks. Many Hispanic people believe that "bad nerves" cause disease when victims become jumpy, irritable, easily startled, overworried, and unable to eat or sleep. Like Italian-Americans, Hispanic-Americans also sometimes attribute disease to the "evil eye."

But perhaps the best-known ethnic remedy is chicken soup, prescribed by Jewish-American grand-mothers for whatever ails you. Modern scientists now attest that "Jewish penicillin" is chock-full of healing nutrients. But how did Grandma know back then?

Between 1880 and 1930 more than two million Jews left Eastern Europe for America. Although their healing traditions varied, it is possible to see distinctive themes in American-Jewish health lore, such as emphasis on diet as a source of health. Names also have great signif-icance in Judaism. Thus, the name of a dangerously sick person, especially a child, might be changed in an attempt to deceive the Angel of Death. Another way Jews have tried to cheat the angel is to symbolically "sell" a sick child to a couple with healthy children. Or the parents of a sick child might visit the graves of beloved relatives and ask for their assistance.

The world is full of people who base their lives on such traditional healing techniques. And even if we don't understand or appreciate those traditions, the fact is that many have produced miraculous cures for thou-sands upon thousands of people. What can we learn by studying the world's mysterious healing secrets? That medicine is indeed a mystery in itself.

Anxiety

Anxiety is the body's and mind's approach to a dangerous or distressing situation. Everyone experiences some degree of anxiety at some time. However, anxiety can occur persistently, often triggered by vague notions of a threat, and interfere with normal activities. When this happens, it's called an anxiety disorder. Symptoms may include irritability, difficulty concentrating, and muscle tension, particularly in the head, neck, and back. Conventional medicine aims to relieve symptoms of persistent anxiety with drug therapy and to treat any underlying disorders or conflicts with psychotherapy.

Repeat yourself. Select a word or sound that is pleasing to you, and say it over and over again to yourself with your eyes closed. In India, devotees of meditation call this a mantra. Weirdly enough, the word doesn't have to mean anything. It can be complete gibberish, but if you chant it long enough, you'll calm down anyway.

Swallow some poison. Popular homeopathic remedies for anxiety include aconite and arsenicum, which are highly toxic. But in homeopathy, doses are so diluted that a chemist might not be able to detect any trace of the main ingredient. Nonetheless, homeopathic medicines seem to produce desired results for thousands of people. See a homeopath, or check your local drugstore, which may stock ready-made homeopathic remedies for anxiety.

Follow the Pied Piper's lead. Legend has it that the Pied Piper of storybook fame lured the rats away from Hamelin by enticing them with valerian (*Valeriana officinalis*), an herb whose pungent odor

KARMIC CONNECTION

According to Tibetan Buddhists, the anxiety you experience in this life may be linked to behaviors from a past life, known as karma. Tibetan medicine's diagnosis of disease also takes into account an individual's karma. And because all actions are said to occur under the influence of a mental state, the fundamental causes of disease are considered to be emotional afflictions, such as desire, anger, and ignorance.

These three mental states are seen as the actual causes of diseases. Factors such as an unbalanced diet, inappropriate behavior, climate, and harmful influences (such as spirits and inauspicious days) are considered secondary causes; they create the potential for negative actions in past lives to produce illness in the present.

The activity of the mind, either in past lives or in the present, lays the foundation for disturbances of the body's system.

reminds many people of dirty socks. Nonetheless, valerian tea is one of the plant world's most potent sedatives.

Sniff a sprig... of lavender (*Lavandula angustifolia*), that is. Aromatherapists say the essential oil produced by this lovely garden plant works wonders to ease jangled nerves.

Squeeze your thumb. Practitioners of *jin shin jyutsu*, a Japanese touch therapy based on the principles of acupuncture, link various emotions with each finger. Worry is said to be the domain of the thumb. Press it gently until you feel yourself relaxing.

Breathe easy with the Bible. Anxious Amish folks sometimes retire to a quiet spot and read the 23rd Psalm. Then they close their eyes and breathe deeply, allowing the psalm's wisdom to soothe them.

Watch your worries go up in smoke. Indians in Mexico and the southwestern United States burn rosemary (*Rosmarinus officinalis*) to drive out evil spirits and purify a person who's suffering from anxiety. Inhale the woody aroma from a burning sprig or from rosemary incense to ease your anxiety.

Veg out. Some people in Indiana relieve anxiety by eating two cups of raw or cooked onions and celery with every meal for a week or two.

Arthritis

Arthritis is a painful disease of the joints. Osteo-arthritis and rheumatoid arthritis are two major types. With osteoarthritis, which often affects the hips, knees, feet, and spine, the joint cartilage deteriorates over time. With rheumatoid arthritis, the membranes lining the joints become inflamed, limiting the joints' range of motion. The body's immune system attacking its own tissues is the most likely cause of rheumatoid arthritis. Because no conventional cure is available, allopathic (modern) medicine's treatment for arthritis focuses on relieving symptoms, which may include swelling, tenderness, pain, and stiffness in one or more joints; limited movement; red, hot, or burning skin over the joints; and even decreased appetite, weight loss, fever, and exhaustion. The typical treatment program consists of drug therapy, exercise, and rest.

Let your mind do some mending. It's actually possible to "think" away pain, although no scientist could tell you why. Your attitude toward your disease, as well as your level of emotional stress and your ability to deal with it, are significant factors in how arthritis will affect you. The hopeful news is that you have control over these factors. Numerous mind-body techniques can help ease arthritis pain, improve range of motion, facilitate sleep, and strengthen your immune system. These include creative visualization, guided imagery, progressive relaxation, support groups, self-hypnosis, and meditation. Your doctor or local hospital may be able to direct you to mind-body resources in your area.

Have your *qi* released. Chinese physicians say arthritis may result from energy, or *qi*, that is blocked. Acupuncture treatments, they say, can restore the energy flow. In addition to stimulating your *qi* with needles placed on "energy points" throughout your body, a Chinese physician is also likely to prescribe an herbal formula tailored to your specific needs.

Indulge in celery. British and German immigrants to America treated rheumatic pain by eating raw or cooked celery seeds (*Apium graveolens*) or large amounts of the celery plant. Eating celery may seem like an unlikely fixative, but there may be something to it, since the custom is still practiced in some parts of the United States.

Try some Native American aspirin. American Indians and early colonists alike used herbs such as white willow (*Salix alba*) and wintergreen (*Gaultheria procumbens*) to control pain. What is truly mysterious is that these plants contain a compound similar to aspirin—a drug that wasn't even invented until the 19th century. (How could they have known?) Aspirin was developed as a less-toxic substitute for methyl-salicylate, a substance that comes from the wintergreen plant; wintergreen was used by Native Americans to treat headache and rheumatic pain. Aspirinlike compounds are also contained in the herbs black cohosh (*Cimicifuga racemosa*), black haw (*Viburnum prunifolium*), and pip-sissewa (*Chimaphila umbellata*).

Put a potato in your pocket. That's what some Appalachian arthritis patients do. Some say that for the remedy to work, the potato must be carried in the right pants pocket. Others say only an Irish potato will do. Strange? Of course. But it may just work—if you believe it will. Any doctor will tell you that the so-called placebo effect has cured countless patients who were given sugar pills but believed they were taking potent medicines.

Count on copper. Wearing a copper bracelet also produces magical cures for some arthritis patients. All in the mind? Maybe, maybe not. A 1976 study found that arthritis patients who wore copper bracelets suffered fewer symptoms than those who wore aluminum bracelets colored to look like copper.

Lie down with the dogs. In Mexico and in the southwest United States, people with arthritis are advised to sleep nestled against a canine. Perhaps the warmth from the mutt brings relief to aching arthritic joints. In some cultures, people believe the disease passes from the person to the animal. You'll find that odd—but apparently popular—belief in some African-

THE HEALING POWER OF AMULETS

How could your arthritis be helped by wearing a copper bracelet or carrying a potato in your pocket? Science can't say. Yet people in every corner of the world have used amulets to ward off illness or to banish it when it strikes.

Amulets are objects said to have spiritual power. Practitioners of folk medicine believe there is a strong link between the spiritual and material, as well as the mental and physical. Amulets are said to protect against harm or to help obtain something good. Amulets have been used to ward off fire, violence, witchcraft, lightning, disease, evil spirits, or anything dangerous and undesirable. Amulets also are thought to attract good luck, health, love, success, or supernatural powers.

Amulets come in many forms. A rabbit's foot and a horseshoe are two that come to mind. In India one of the most powerful amulets is made by gluing together bits of wood from ten different types of sacred trees and then wrapping the bundle with gold wire.

Amulets can also be made of plants. Garlic is widely reputed to repel evil forces. Metals and stones are used as well. And amulets can be devised from written materials, ranging from magical charms written on pieces of paper and sealed in a small sack to entire books.

American communities, as well as in North Carolina, Kentucky, Indiana, Illinois, Texas, Kansas, and Nebraska.

Try traditional seeds of relief. Chinese folk healers recommend eating sesame seeds, about half an ounce a day, to relieve arthritis discomfort. Grind them in a coffee grinder, and sprinkle them on your food at mealtime.

Muster up some mustard. Mustard may seem an odd or magical arthritis remedy, but employing so-called counterirritants to ease pain is a technique of folk healers throughout Europe, Asia, and the Appalachia area of the United States even today. Counterirritants are substances that irritate and inflame the skin over a painful area, perhaps drawing circulation to the area or perhaps simply providing a distraction for the patient with arthritis pain. One of the oldest counterirritants is the mustard plaster. Crush the seeds of white or brown mustard (*Brassica* spp.), or grind them in a coffee grinder. Moisten with vinegar, then sprinkle on flour to thicken. Spread the mixture on a cloth, and place the poultice—mustard side down—on the skin, leaving it on for no longer than twenty minutes. Then remove the plaster and wash the affected area thoroughly.

Pepper your pain away. Cayenne pepper is another counterirritant used in China and in the Southwest and Midwest regions of the United States.

Steep one ounce cayenne (*Capsicum annuum*) in one quart rubbing alcohol. Let stand for three weeks, shaking the bottle each day. Then, using a cloth, apply the lotion to the affected area for twenty minutes. Wipe clean.

Bites & Stings

When bees, wasps, and other insects bite or sting you, they may release a poisonous venom that produces pain, swelling, redness, itching, or burning. Most people recover from a bee or wasp sting in a couple of hours. But about three percent of the population develops an allergic reaction called anaphylaxis, in which painful hives erupt and swelling blocks airways, leading to circulatory collapse and even death. Conventional medicine alleviates symptoms of common stings and bites with drugs, ointments, and lotions.

Smother it with onion. A homegrown Amish remedy for bee stings is to apply a freshly cut onion (*Allium cepa*). Hold the onion slice on the wound for at least ten minutes, then discard.

Smear on some baking supplies. Who'd have thought that a couple of kitchen staples could take the bite out of a bee sting? Well, someone, at some time, came up with this traditional folk remedy. Mix one tablespoon each of vinegar and baking soda. Apply the paste, and leave it on the sting as long as possible. Add more, if necessary.

Try some tobacco. But don't smoke it or chew it, 'cause that stuff can kill you. Instead, apply it to bug bites and stings in a traditional poultice. Maya Indians used wild tobacco (*Nicotiana rustica, N. glauca*), moistened with saliva, to treat bee stings. Mysteriously, the unlikely remedy was also employed by the Six Nations, a league of Indians extending from the Hudson River to Lake Erie, although there is no evidence that those people ever had any contact with the Central American Mayas. In some parts of Appalachia today, tobacco poultices are still used to heal bee, hornet, yellow jacket, wasp, and spider bites and stings.

Do as the Seventh Day Adventists do. Seventh Day Adventists don't barbecue burgers, but they do use charcoal to heal insect bites. Charcoal, they say, draws out the poison. Wet as much charcoal (not the kind that contains lighter fluid) as needed to cover your wound. Place the paste directly over the wound, and cover it with a clean cloth. Replace the poultice every ten to fifteen minutes until you obtain relief.

Keep a Gypsy potion ready. Gypsies wash stings and bites with vinegar to stop itching and relieve pain. Here's a favorite recipe you can prepare ahead of time: Seal a handful of thyme (*Thymus vulgaris*) in a bottle of vinegar, and place it in the sun. Leave it for one cycle of the moon, shaking the bottle mornings and evenings. After an additional half cycle of the moon, crush seven garlic cloves, add them to the potion, and reseal. At the end of the second lunar cycle, strain the liquid and store it in a sealed bottle. When you get an insect bite or sting, wash the wound with the potion.

Bladder & Kidney Problems

The urinary bladder can become infected with bacteria that normally inhabit the intestinal tract. Bladder infections are much more common in women than in men because a woman's urethra—the passage that leads from the bladder to the outside of the body—is much shorter than a man's, thus allowing bacteria to travel to the bladder more easily. Bladder infections can recur again and again, and the kidneys and other parts of the urinary tract may also become infected. Symptoms may include a burning and stinging sensation when urinating; cloudy, bloody, or unusual-smelling urine; a frequent urge to urinate that produces only small amounts of urine; and pain in the lower abdomen or back. Conventional medicine typically relies on drug therapy, including antibiotics.

 Get your spine adjusted. It may seem odd that manipulating your spine could help heal a bladder

THE THREE TIBETAN HUMORS

Tibetans believe the body is regulated by three types of energy, called humors. The humors—wind, bile, and phlegm—perform various functions within the body. Disease results when humors become unbalanced. So the job of a Tibetan physician is to restore harmony to the humors.

infection. But chiropractors reportedly clear up bladder problems by rebalancing patients' vertebrae.

Look to the trees. Aromatherapists say bladder infections respond well to essential oils of pine (*Pinus* spp.), sandalwood (*Santalum album*), cedarwood (*Cedrus* spp.), tea tree (*Melaleuca alternifolia*), and juniper (*Juniperus communis*). The oils can be used (diluted) in body compresses, massages (mixed with warm oil), or warm sitz baths.

Go berry picking. For centuries, the Amish and other groups have drunk the juice of cranberries to relieve the pain of urinary infections. Scientists only recently discovered that cranberry juice indeed has compounds that help the urinary tract heal. Native Americans also taught Pennsylvania Germans to make a healing tea from corn silk (*Zea mays*). To make the tea, fill a one-quart jar with boiling water and about two-thirds cup of corn silk. Steep until cool. Strain and drink one cup three times a day for seven to ten days.

◉ **Try a spoonful of sugar.** Gypsies in Spain added sugar or honey to teas when treating urinary tract infections. Try adding some to a noncaffeinated tea.

◉ **Have your tummy touched.** Acupressurists say that stimulating points along the stomach meridian may help to alleviate bladder infections.

Burns & Sunburn

A superficial burn is a first-degree burn, typical of a simple sunburn. A second-degree burn penetrates deeper into the skin and is usually accompanied by blisters. Third-degree burns involve deep tissue destruction. Serious burns, large burns, and burns on the face or hands should be treated by a physician, but minor burns can be treated at home. Symptoms include red, swollen, inflamed skin and, perhaps, some blistering. Conventional treatment for simple burns involves cooling the tissues as quickly as possible to reduce inflammation and blistering, and then applying soothing ointment. (If you have any doubt about the severity of a burn, forego home remedies and see a doctor.)

◉ **Do as Seventh Day Adventists do.** Seventh Day Adventists somehow discovered long ago that adding baking soda to your bath can help ease the discomfort of sunburn. To test it yourself, fill a tub with lukewarm water, add a cup of baking soda, and soak for thirty to sixty minutes. When you're done, let your skin dry naturally. Don't chafe it with a towel.

Seek relief from Mother Nature's medicine. Every culture in the world has used the aloe plant's soothing sap to treat all types of minor burns—even without scientific evidence to prove its effectiveness. Slice the leaf down the middle, and rub the goo on your burn. Or make a lotion by adding two ounces of fresh aloe vera sap to eight ounces of extra virgin olive oil.

Take a tip from Native American medicine. American Indians, as well as Appalachian residents, wash burns in tobacco tea, and Indiana farmers apply chewing tobacco. To make the tea, remove the tobacco from a pack of cigarettes and add to one quart water. Boil until the volume is reduced to one pint. Strain the tea and let it cool to room temperature. Then wash the burn with the tea as often as necessary.

Try a time-tested technique known from India to Indiana. In New England, Indiana, North Carolina—and as far away as India—burn victims have found relief by applying a poultice of grated raw potatoes. Hold the mash in place with a cloth, and change the dressing every hour or two until the burn is healed.

Reach for sweet relief. Chinese immigrants put honey on burns, then cover the wound with sterile gauze. If you want to try this remedy, be sure to cool the burn under clean, cool water first. Also, change the bandage three to four times a day.

Find comfort with lavender (*Lavandula angustifolia*). This herb has been used in medicinal potions for centuries. Modern-day aromatherapists believe that easing the pain of burns is amongst its benefits. And some modern research suggests that it may have antiseptic properties as well. Aromatherapists advise you to add five drops of lavender oil to one pint of water, stirring well to disperse the oil. Apply to burns with a clean cloth. Leave the compress on the wound for several minutes, then resoak the cloth and apply at least two more times.

Cold, Flu & Cough

The common cold is aptly named. It is so common, in fact, that all human beings from every region of the globe experience it at one time or another during their lives. A simple common cold is a collection of familiar symptoms signaling an infection of the upper respiratory tract, which includes the nose, throat, and sinuses. At least five major categories of viruses cause colds. One of these groups, and perhaps the most common, the rhinoviruses, includes a minimum of 100 different viruses.

Although we often say "colds and flu" in the same breath, influenza is a very different disease from the common cold. The influenza virus takes up residence mainly in the throat and bronchial tract. If you have the flu, you usually have a fever, and a fever is not usually present in a cold. The fever usually passes within three days, but the fatigue, muscle aches, and cough that result from the flu can linger for weeks.

Follow the plains. For centuries, Plains Indians used purple coneflower, or echinacea (*Echinacea angustifolia, Echinacea purpurea*), as a remedy for colds and flu. Today, it's the best-selling herbal remedy in the country. Several studies suggest that echinacea activates the immune system, the body's natural agent of healing, but scientists don't completely understand how. You can purchase a tincture of echinacea at a health-food store, herb shop, or drugstore. At the first sign of a cold or flu, take one teaspoon of the tincture every hour for three hours. If the infection persists, take one dropperful of the tincture every three hours, even if you're taking other cold medications.

Eat like an ancient Egyptian. The recommendation to take garlic (*Allium sativum*) for colds comes from New England, the American Southwest, and all the way from China. Garlic has been used for colds, bronchial problems, and fevers in cultures throughout the world since the dawn of written medical history. Even the ancient Egyptians used it to treat cough and fever. Blend three cloves of garlic in a blender with a little water. (The clove must be cut or crushed in order

Folk traditions often advise a cold or flu sufferer to sip hot, fragrant teas. Most herbs used to treat colds—elder (*Sambucus* spp.), ginger (*Zingiber officinale*), yarrow (*Achillea millefolium*), mint (*Mentha* spp.), thyme (*Thymus vulgaris*), lemon balm (*Melissa officinalis*), catnip (*Nepeta cataria*), garlic (*Allium sativum*), onion *(Allium cepa),* and mustard (*Brassica* spp.)—contain aromatic oils that have recently been shown to produce antibacterial, antiviral, antifungal, and anti-inflammatory actions. The oils escape with the steam of hot tea. The steam delivers the oil's constituents directly to the surface of the mucous membranes, where they attack the invading organism causing the cold.

to release its constituents.) If you want, add half a lemon, skin and all, to the garlic. Put the contents in a cup and fill the cup with boiling water. Let steep for five minutes, inhaling the fragrance. Strain, add honey, and drink the entire cup in sips. Do this two to three times a day while you have a cold or flu, or once a day to prevent infection during epidemics.

Take advantage of a rural remedy. Onions, cousins to garlic, have also been used to treat colds in virtually every folk tradition in North America, whether eaten raw, roasted, or boiled; taken in the form of teas, milk, or wine; worn in a sock or in a bag around the neck; or applied to the chest as a poultice. Wild onions have been used for the same purpose by Native American tribes in every region of the country. Using onions to treat colds persists today in the folk medicine of New England, upstate New York, North Carolina, Appalachia, Indiana, and within Chinese communities throughout North America. Perhaps because the onion's pungent aroma seems to cut through even the stuffiest nose, cold sufferers have been drawn to the bulb. And now, even modern science seems to confirm that the plant has anti-infective properties. To see for yourself, cut up one large onion and simmer in a covered pot for twenty minutes. Drink a cup of the tea three to four times daily when you have a cold or flu.

Follow sage advice from New England. Some residents of New England, North Carolina, and Indiana recommend hot sage (*Salvia officinalis*) tea to "break up" a cold. They say sage is especially good for sore throats that often accompany colds. (*See* Sore Throat.) Place one teaspoon of sage in a cup and fill with boiling water. Cover and let steep for ten minutes. Strain, add a little lemon and honey, and drink. Repeat three to four times a day for as long as you have a cold.

Do as the Romans. The contemporary folk traditions of New England and Indiana call for drinking hot lemonade during a cold or flu, but the practice is at least as old as the ancient Romans. What made our ancestors turn to a lemon for relief is unknown.

To make this time-tested potion, place one chopped, whole lemon—skin, pulp, and all—in a pot, and add one cup of boiling water. While letting the mixture steep for five minutes, inhale the fumes. Then strain and drink. Do this at the onset of a cold, and repeat three to four times a day for the duration of the cold.

Test the wisdom of Hippocrates. Inhaling the fumes of vinegar is a cold remedy as old as ancient Greece. Yes, even the Greek physician Hippocrates recommended the treatment for coughs and respiratory infections. In a jar, pour half a cup of boiling water over half a cup of vinegar. Gently inhale the steam, but be careful not to burn yourself.

Turn to salt. It's unclear who figured out that sniffing salt water could ease nasal congestion, nor how they happened upon the discovery. The remedy is part of New England and Indiana folk medicine and is now often recommended by conventional medical doctors. Ayurvedic physicians in India even use a special pot, called a neti, to make the process easier. To help yourself breathe easier, put a quarter teaspoon of salt in a glass of hot or warm water, and sniff some of the water. Do this after being exposed to someone with a cold or flu, or at the first sign of infection. Repeat every three to four hours while suffering from a cold.

Try buttering yourself up. Adding butter to hot tea is a remedy used in the high altitudes of Nepal and Tibet to prevent colds. Add one tablespoon of butter to a cup of hot tea. Let the butter melt, so that it forms a thin layer across the top of the tea. Stir and drink. New Englanders use a similar technique—adding butter to hot water—to treat colds.

Look to the mountains for relief. Yak meat clears phlegm, according to Tibetan wisdom. Fortunately for those of us who don't know any yak farmers, there are other foods recommended for phlegm disorders. They include mutton, meat of wild carnivorous animals, fish, honey, warm porridge, yogurt, whey, strong beer, and boiled water.

Depression

Clinical depression is an illness that causes a person's mood and behavior to change for long periods. Depression is characterized mainly by feelings of sadness, irritability, or indifference. Depression may result from a chemical imbalance in the brain, and episodes can be triggered by a traumatic event, prolonged stress, and other factors. Symptoms may include lack of interest in hobbies or other activities that once were enjoyable; changes in weight, appetite, or sleeping; feelings of guilt, worthlessness, or hopelessness; and confusion and fatigue. Conventional medicine treats depression with drugs and psychotherapy.

Take a dose of sadness. It sounds ironic, but practitioners of homeopathy treat depression with highly diluted natural substances that would cause symptoms of depression if given in full strength to a healthy person. Some homeopathic remedies are even designed to help a depressed person open up and express his feelings. See a homeopathic physician for evaluation.

Say "OM." Take advantage of the wisdom of Indian healing: Regular practice of yoga and some breath-

✺ MYSTERIOUS ST. JOHN'S WORT ✺

You've probably heard that scientists have validated the centuries-old practice of using St. John's wort (*Hypericum perforatum*) to treat depression. Seems the plant indeed has mood-lifting properties. In fact, it worked as well in some studies as expensive pharmaceutical drugs. Exactly how and why, no one knows for sure. But thousands of people in the United States and Europe take it every day.

The Amish use St. John's wort to treat depression, too. But they don't consume the plant. They hang it over the barn door or house door to keep out witches and their spells. Thus, they believe, they prevent depression and other illnesses from striking their families.

ing exercises can instill energy and confidence and reduce stress. Check your yellow pages or contact your local hospital to find out about yoga and other stress-reduction classes.

Get to the point of trouble. Acupuncturists consider depression to result from a blockage of *qi*, the body's vital energy force. Acupuncture aims to rebalance the flow of *qi* by stimulating energy points in specific areas. An acupuncturist would likely stimulate points along the heart meridian to ease the symptoms of depression.

Count your blessings. That's the advice of the Amish, who rely on faith, Bible scripture, and community support to deal with depression. An Amish elder might recommend that you do something good for someone else, make a list of all the good things in your life, and pray, according to your faith.

Try a hands-on remedy. One study found that thirty minutes of massage a day effectively reduced depression and anxiety in hospital patients. Could there be something magical in the human touch? Test it for yourself and decide.

Stop and smell the flowers. It's an old cliché. But there may actually be an antidepressant effect from inhaling certain fragrances. The aroma of flowers such as orange blossom (*Citrus aurantium*), jasmine

(*Jasminum officinalis*), and ylang ylang (*Cananga odorata*) appears to alleviate symptoms of depression.

◉ **Eat your oatmeal.** At the turn of the 20th century, physicians widely prescribed oats (*Avena sativa*) as a remedy for depression. Exactly why is unclear, but it's unlikely to hurt you to give it a try.

◉ **Dissolve your worries.** Seventh Day Adventists take a "neutral bath" to relieve depression. They soak in water kept within a degree or two of body temperature for twenty to forty minutes. Why the temperature should be "neutral" is unclear, but perhaps it's the *lack* of heat or cold that helps them regain balance.

Diabetes

Diabetes mellitus is a disorder that prevents the body from effectively converting carbohydrates (sugars and starches) into energy. Insulin-dependent (Type I) diabetes occurs when the pancreas gland stops producing insulin, a hormone that helps in the conversion process. Non-insulin-dependent (Type II) diabetes happens when the body doesn't properly use the insulin it has. Symptoms may include constant thirst, frequent urination, fatigue, muscle weakness, or blurred vision. There is no cure for diabetes, so doctors try to manage the disease with drug therapy, insulin injections, and lifestyle changes. (Keep in mind that diabetes is nothing to mess with; it can cause permanent damage in the body. So be sure to discuss any alternative therapies with your doctor first.)

Be willful. Some people with diabetes can improve their symptoms by "willing" themselves to get better. Biofeedback and relaxation techniques can teach diabetics how to reduce stress. That's key, since stress hormones can increase blood sugar levels.

Enlist the help of your subconscious. Hypnosis can offer the subconscious mind suggestions that the body needs less insulin.

Strike a pose. Regular practice of yoga poses and breathing exercises can improve blood sugar levels

TINKLING IN TIBET

Diabetics often test their urine to determine their blood sugar levels. In Tibet, doctors examine a patient's urine to determine if there are imbalances in any of the "humors" that are thought to control disease. Changes observed in a patient's urine immediately after it has been stirred indicate the nature of the patient's humoral disturbance. Tibetan doctors then treat the condition with natural medicines tailored to individual needs.

in some diabetics. It may sound odd, but it likely has to do with reducing stress levels in the body.

Consider an Asian therapy plan. To treat diabetes, Chinese medicine uses herbs, acupuncture, calorie-restricted diets, and mind-body exercises, including *qi gong* (chee gung). To find out more, contact a qualified practitioner of Chinese medicine who has experience in treating diabetes. And stay in touch with your regular physician.

Give yourself a metal. Taking chromium picolinate, a mineral supplement, has enabled many Type II diabetics to lower the amount of prescription medicine they need. Discuss the possible benefits of this supplement with your doctor.

Let your feet do the healing. Sounds incredible, but reflexologists say massaging certain points on the feet can reduce blood glucose levels in patients with Type II diabetes. Because people with diabetes tend to have poor circulation and may have nerve damage in the feet, see a trained reflexologist who has experience working with diabetics if you want to try this remedy.

Digestive Problems

Ancient healers of Greece, India, and China believed that the digestive tract was the root of the tree of good health. If the digestive tract were healthy, they reasoned, the body could readily absorb muscle- and bone-building nutrients from foods.

Irregular or improperly functioning digestion can, indeed, cause or contribute to disease anywhere in the body. Symptoms of digestive problems may include flatulence or belching; nausea; pain in the stomach; offensive breath; constipation; lethargy or depression; and unusual food cravings. Conventional medicine often fails to diagnose digestive problems, and many people resort to over-the-counter remedies for indigestion, constipation, and nausea.

Take your mother's advice. When you were little, your mother probably gave you a glass of ginger ale when your tummy was upset. It's a remedy favored by moms in New England, Appalachia, and around the world, including India, China, Saudi Arabia, and the Caribbean. Ginger (*Zingiber officinale*) does help to settle your stomach. But how did all of those moms know?

To be most effective, you must use real ginger ale, not just ginger-flavored soda. Or, make ginger tea. Stir half a teaspoon of ground ginger into one cup of hot water, and steep about five minutes. Drink up to three cups a day.

Avail yourself of an Arabian remedy. Chew caraway seeds (*Carum carvi*) to relieve gas and ease digestion. It's a remedy that's been used for centuries in cultures around the world, particularly among the Arabs.

In India and the Middle East, thoughtful hosts pass a small bowl of caraway or fennel (*Foeniculum vulgare*) seeds for guests to nibble after sumptuous meals. It's not clear why it works, but plenty of diners swear by it.

Keep it topical. Seventh Day Adventists apply hot compresses to the abdomen after heavy meals. Presumably, the heat attracts circulation to the area, thus improving digestion, although the remedy may first have been used simply because it feels soothing.

Remember castor oil. In a trance, psychic Edgar Cayce advised applying castor oil to the stomach. There's no scientific evidence to support the seer's claim, but hundreds of people swore they found digestive relief after trying the remedy. Now it's a standard treatment in North American schools for naturopathic physicians. Castor oil, taken internally, is a strong laxative. Applied to the body in a compress or pack, however, it produces no such effect yet somehow improves digestion.

Use your nose to aid your stomach. Merely inhaling the scent of certain essential oils, according to aromatherapists, can improve digestion and eliminate gas. Useful digestive herb oils include black pepper (*Piper nigrum*), clary sage (*Salvia sclarea*), juniper berry (*Juniperus communis*), lemongrass (*Cymbopogon citratus*), peppermint (*Mentha piperita*), rosemary (*Rosmarinus officinalis*), and thyme (*Thymus vulgaris*).

SPICE UP YOUR LIFE

A variety of plants appear to work on the digestive system. For example, to stimulate digestion, you can try carminative herbs such as anise (*Pimpinella anisum*), basil (*Ocimum basilicum*), caraway (*Carum carvi*), coriander (*Coriandrum sativum*), and fennel (*Foeniculum vulgare)*. Rosemary is said to improve food absorption, and peppermint treats irritable bowel syndrome. Basil overcomes nausea from chemotherapy or radiation treatments, even when conventional antinausea drugs have failed. And lemongrass is used in Brazil, the Caribbean, and Southeast Asia to relieve nervous stomachs. How these herbs work is a mystery.

Carminative herbs often are combined with bitter herbs in formulas. In folk medicine and traditional herbalism, bitter tonics are frequently prescribed to stimulate appetite. Bitter tonics include wormwood (*Artemisia absinthium*), chamomile (*Matricaria recutita*), goldenseal (*Hydrastis canadensis*), Oregon grape root (*Mahonia aquifolium*), gentian (*Gentiana lutea*), and boneset (*Eupatorium perfoliatum*).

Warm up your engine. Tibetan physicians believe an overabundance of "phlegm" leads to a decrease in "digestive heat." The result is indigestion. To increase digestive heat, they prescribe pomegranate (*Punica* *granatum*). And fennel (*Foeniculum vulgare*) is thought to improve the appetite.

Ear Problems

The ear can become infected in any of its three parts—the inner ear, the middle ear, or the outer ear. Infections most commonly occur in the middle and outer ear. These may develop when viruses or bacteria in the nose or throat travel to the ear through the Eustachian tube, which connects the three organs. Ear infections are more likely to afflict children than adults. Symptoms may include pain and inflammation. Conventional medicine treats the condition with antibiotics and other drugs.

Give basil a new job. Though basil (*Ocimum basilicum*) is better known for spicing up spaghetti sauce, in Spanish-speaking parts of the United States, as well as in Mexico and Central America, many people use the fragrant herb to cure earaches. Place one ounce of basil leaves in one pint of vegetable oil. Cover tightly and let sit in a warm place for two weeks, shaking the jar daily. Strain and reserve the oil. Then, put six to eight drops of the oil into the ear canal four times a day.

Prepare a Spanish-born remedy. Another unusual remedy derives from cloves. Cloves (*Syzgium aromaticum*) were brought by Arab traders from Southeast

Asia to Spain. Settlers then took the cure to America. To use this remedy, grind half an ounce of clove in a coffee grinder and add it to half a pint of olive oil. Cover and keep in a warm place for three or four days, shaking the bottle each day. Strain and put six to eight drops of the oil in each ear.

Eye Problems

Inflammations of the eye can be painful and produce redness, swelling, and irritation. Conjunctivitis, or pinkeye, is an inflammation of the conjunctiva, the delicate membrane that lines the inner curve of the eyelid and covers the exposed surface of the eye. The infection results from disease-causing microorganisms, such as bacteria, fungi, and viruses. Eye inflammation also may be caused by allergies, chemicals, dust, smoke, and foreign objects that become lodged in the eye. Conventional treatment varies according to cause and symptoms. Doctors may prescribe antibiotics, steroids, or soothing eyedrops.

How about a spot of tea? Tea is a common eye remedy, from Appalachia to India and other Asian countries. It's easy if you use black- or green-tea bags. Prepare tea according to directions. Then place the tea bag on your closed eye for 15 minutes. Repeat as needed. Meanwhile, sip away.

Try a remedy that smells sweet. A rose is a rose is a . . . cure for infected eyes, as they might say in Spanish- and Arabic-speaking communities. Go out to the garden and pick roses that are free of pesticides and other chemicals. Place a handful of petals in a jar and add one pint of boiling water. Cover well to retain the aromatic oils and let stand until the water has cooled to room temperature. Strain, then soak a clean cloth with the liquid and place on the closed eye.

Apply an Incan poultice. This unlikely cure comes from the Incas. The Incas cultivated potatoes as a food and medicine, and one medical use included eye conditions. Remove the skin from a whole raw potato and grate finely. Place the grated potato in a clean cloth and fold to make a poultice. Apply the poultice to your eye for 15 minutes.

Use a plant that has "eyes." Europeans have long used the lowly weed eyebright (*Euphrasia officinalis*) to treat conjunctivitis and other eye infections. Eyebright's flowers look like little yellow eyes and, apparently, this resemblance sparked some ingenious individual to try it as an eye remedy. European colonists brought the remedy with them to the New World. You'll find it today in parts of Appalachia. Place one tablespoon of eyebright leaves in one pint of hot water. Cover and steep for ten minutes. Strain and apply the liquid with a clean cloth, while sipping a cup of the tea. Do this twice a day.

Give yourself flowers. Many Asian-Americans know that chrysanthemum blossoms (*Chrysanthemum indicum flos*) make a great remedy for tired,

WARDING OFF THE EVIL EYE

There is a widespread belief, especially among Italian Americans, that the "evil eye" can cause disease. People with the power to evoke the evil eye may do so intentionally or unintentionally, usually because they are envious or jealous of a person. Children and pregnant women, who are naturally vulnerable, are considered prime targets for this type of curse.

Thus, you must pinch a child's cheek if you praise him. Or a person who has complimented a child may try to abort unintentional envy by spitting and saying, "I mean no harm."

To cure a sickness caused by the evil eye, the victim seeks out a healer, usually a woman who has been handed down her healing secrets. She may advise the victim to wear a charm or amulet in the shape of an eye, heart, hand, or horn; eat garlic; or carry written copies of religious texts.

Red and blue are favorite colors for warding off evil-eye sicknesses. Christians and Jews in North and South America attach red ribbons to children's clothing or hair. In Europe and Mediterranean countries, blue stones are used as charms to deflect the malicious power of the evil eye.

aching eyes. The Chinese and Japanese place a large handful of flowers in a pot and add one quart of boiling water. This is covered and steeped for ten minutes, and then strained. The wet flowers are wrapped in a clean cloth. Then, the poultice is placed on the eye while the patient sips the tea.

Calm them with chamomile. Aromatherapists recommend a chamomile cure for tired eyes. Steep two chamomile (*Matricaria recutita*) tea bags in a few tablespoons of hot water. Allow the bags to cool somewhat. Then lie down and place a tea bag over each eye. Cover the poultices with a soft cloth.

Try a Tibetan tip for stressed out eyes. In Tibet, a tea made of fennel (*Foeniculum vulgare*) is used to soothe tired, irritated eyes.

Fatigue

Fatigue results from physical or mental exhaustion and may be accompanied by overwhelming feelings of weariness, lack of energy or enthusiasm, and a number of other symptoms. Fatigue itself is a symptom of a vast number of diseases and disorders, as well as an ailment in its own right. Conventional doctors recommend rest and a regimen of good nutrition and exercise, as well as treating any illnesses that may be contributing to the condition.

Find yourself a chicken. A traditional American remedy for fatigue is to eat an egg every day, although exactly why or how this would help is unclear.

Swallow a bitter pill. Bitters are the 19th-century remedy that some German physicians still prescribe today. Bitter tonics are made from plants with a strong bitter flavor, but the medicines are not strong themselves. In fact, many act as mild sedatives. And yet, they've been documented to cure fatigue. The most famous bitter herbs in North America are goldthread (*Coptis trifolia*), goldenseal (*Hydrastis canadensis*), Oregon grape root (*Mahonia aquifolium*), yellow dock (*Rumex crispus*), dandelion root (*Taraxacum officinale*), and betony (*Betonica officinalis*).

Wake up with rosemary. It is said that rosemary (*Rosmarinus officinalis*) can raise energy levels. Add a few sprigs to your bath or sip a cup of rosemary tea. To make tea, steep one teaspoon of rosemary in one cup hot water for fifteen minutes. Drink up to three cups a day.

Get yourself some *Guter Schlof.* That's Amish German for "good sleep." The ever-practical Amish say the best remedy for fatigue is sleep. That's not earth-shattering, of course, but the Amish don't stop there in their prescription for refreshing sleep. They say one hour of sleep before midnight is worth two hours of sleep after the clock strikes twelve (in other words, go to bed earlier rather than sleeping later). Also an Amish belief is that a half-hour afternoon nap is the equivalent of two hours of sleep at night. Another old Amish remedy for fatigue is to sleep with your head pointing north.

⊚ **Get prodded out of your fatigue.** An insufficiency of *qi*, the body's vital force, can cause myriad symptoms, including fatigue, according to practitioners of Chinese medicine. Acupuncture and moxibustion are used to bring energy to deficient organs and systems.

⊚ **Brew a Christmas cure.** Ancient Incas and their modern descendants have brewed a tea from holly (*Ilex guayusa, Ilex paraguariensis*) to cure fatigue. The tea is drunk as a morning eye-opener and to relieve exhaustion after long journeys or heavy labor.

Female Problems

Mild to severe discomfort in the days preceding the monthly menstrual period is common. Symptoms of the condition, known as premenstrual syndrome (PMS), may include painful cramps, bloating, headaches, and emotional upset. When monthly bleeding stops in midlife, menopause sets in and may be accompanied by its own set of uncomfortable symptoms, including hot flashes. Doctors may prescribe drugs, hormones, and over-the-counter remedies to treat menstrual discomfort and the symptoms of menopause.

Call on Mother Nature. Many plants provide relief from menstrual problems, although science can't say why. These include ginger (*Zingiber officinale*), tansy (*Tanacetum vulgare*), juniper (*Juniperus communis*), rosemary (*Rosmarinus officinalis*), basil (*Ocimum basilicum*), thyme (*Thymus vulgaris*), cinnamon (*Cinnamomum zeylanicum*), yarrow (*Achillea millefolium*), chamomile (*Matricaria recutita*), and fennel (*Foeniculum vulgare*). Teas made from the plants may be sipped or used as compresses.

Enlist patchouli for PMS. If you suffer from excessive bloating or swollen breasts as part of premenstrual syndrome (PMS), use the essential oil of patchouli (*Pogostemon cablin*). Another good PMS oil is birch (*Betula lenta*), which relieves pain. For water retention, turn to juniper berry (*Juniperus communis*). And marjoram *(Origanum majorana)* oil can curb PMS headaches. Other oils useful for treating PMS include chamomile, clary sage, geranium, jasmine, neroli, and rose. Add the oils to your bath or mix them with vegetable oil and massage them on your skin.

Look to China. Chinese physicians believe painful menstruation is caused by variations, deficiencies, or stagnation of qi and blood. When *qi*, the vital life force, is more stagnant than blood, PMS symptoms appear. Chinese doctors have had great success in treating PMS with herbs, acupuncture, and moxibustion.

Think bland. If you suffer from PMS, a Chinese physician will also advise you to avoid sweets as well as strong spices, such as hot peppers, and stimulants, such as coffee.

Get down to essentials to ease menopause discomforts. Essential oils of several plants ease symptoms of menopause by balancing estrogen and other hormones. Particularly helpful are cypress (*Cupressus sempervirens*), geranium (*Pelargonium graveoloens*), lavender (*Lavandula angustifolia*), neroli (*Citrus aurantium*), rose (*Rosa* spp.), and clary sage (*Salvia sclarea*). To cool down from a hot flash, try clary sage, lemon (*Citrus limonum*), or peppermint (*Mentha piperita*). Oils to smooth out emotional ups

---

MENOPAUSE BODY OIL

Use this fragrant, soothing oil to chill out after a hot flash.

  6 drops lemon oil
  5 drops geranium oil
  2 drops clary sage oil
  1 drop angelica oil
  1 drop jasmine oil
  2 ounces vegetable oil

Combine all ingredients and store in a tightly capped bottle. Use at least once a day as a massage oil or lotion. Or add two teaspoons to a warm bath, and soak.

---

and downs include chamomile *(Matricaria recutita)*, jasmine *(Jasminum officinalis)*, and neroli. Massage the oils directly on your skin, or add them to bath water.

Fever

The body's normal temperature is around 98.6 degrees Fahrenheit. To qualify as a fever, the temperature usually has to top 100 degrees. A fever is a symptom of infection, such as flu, measles, or tonsillitis, or another ailment, ranging from dehydration to heart attack. Symptoms may accompany fever, including headache, thirst, redness of the face, chills, and mental confusion. Conventional medicine attempts to lower body temperature with over-the-counter medicines, such as aspirin, or to fight infection with antibiotics.

Consider using "hair of the dog." Homeopaths treat a fever by giving you a highly diluted dose of a natural substance that would produce a fever in a healthy person. In addition, a homeopathic physician might ask you questions that seem strange, such as "Does one cheek feel redder or warmer than the other?" or "Does urinating make you feel better?" To top it off, this mysterious type of therapy might call for a prescription made with infinitesimal doses of poisons, such as belladonna and nux vomica.

Ease it with oil. Some essential oils will cool you off. Apply or inhale bergamot (*Citrus bergamia*), chamomile (*Matricaria recutita*), or eucalyptus (*Eucalyptus globulus*).

Find out who your enemies are. Some Hispanics believe fevers result from *mal ojo,* or the evil eye. Symptoms of a curse may include sudden onset of high fever, vomiting, headache, fainting, or convulsions. To diagnose a curse, a healer examines a fresh egg that's broken after being passed over the patient's body. If the egg appears to be cooked, or has the image of an eye, the person is said to have been bewitched. To effect a cure, the perpetrator must be induced to touch the patient as soon as possible.

Reach for sour relief. Hot lemonade is a fever remedy in New England and India—and the ancient Romans used it, too. Pour one cup of boiling water over a blended whole lemon—skin, pulp, and all. Steep the mixture for five minutes, while inhaling the fumes. Then drink one cup at the onset of fever, and repeat three to four times a day while ill.

Slice up some onion. Onions (*Allium cepa*) are a near-universal remedy for fever, although why they should have this effect—especially considering some of the ways they're employed—is truly a mystery. Most American Indians used onions to bring down temperature, and the remedy is still in use in New England, New

SWEATING IT OUT

Sweating is essential to cool the body during a fever. Many traditional folk remedies use herbs for this purpose. These diaphoretic herbs have constituents that, when eaten, increase the blood circulation to the skin, which causes perspiration and ultimately lowers the fever.

Diaphoretic herbs include boneset (*Eupatorium perfoliatum*), catnip (*Nepeta cataria*), cinnamon (*Cinnamomum zeylanicum*), elder (*Sambucus nigra*), ginger (*Zingiber officinale*), mint (*Mentha* spp.), thyme (*Thymus vulgaris*), yarrow (*Achillea millefolium*), lemon balm (*Melissa officinalis*), and garlic (*Allium sativum*).

It is essential to drink plenty of fluids when taking these herbs, however, or dehydration may result. They're most effective when taken as hot teas. After drinking the tea, go to bed, wrap up in warm blankets, and sweat it out. Continue to drink plenty of fluids.

York, North Carolina, parts of Appalachia, Indiana, and even China. Some people recommend placing onion slices on the bottoms of the feet, under the patient's bed, in a sock or bag worn around the patient's neck, or applied to the chest as a poultice. Others prescribe onions raw, roasted, or boiled or added to tea, milk, or even wine.

Get cold feet. Reactive hydrotherapy, a practice taught in North American naturopathic colleges, has its roots in Gypsy lore. Soak cotton socks in cold water, wring them out, and place them on the patient's feet. Cover the cold socks with one or two pairs of warm wool socks and leave in place at least 40 minutes.

Take a tip from Tibet. Tibetan physicians prescribe several herbs for reducing fever, including white sandalwood (*Santalum album*), fennel (*Foeniculum vulgare*), and scute (*Scutellaria baicalensis*).

Foot Problems

The most common foot problem is athlete's foot. Athlete's foot is a fungal infection that often takes hold as a result of poor foot hygiene (failing to keep the feet clean and dry) or a weakness of the immune system. Conventional medicine prescribes antifungal creams and ointments, as well as improvements in hygiene. Another common foot problem is cold feet, for which conventional medicine has few if any fixes. Keep in mind that if you have diabetes or circulation problems, you should always see a doctor for treatment of foot problems rather than rely on home remedies.

Dance in the garden. Sounds silly, but some people have cured foot conditions by crushing herbs and rubbing them over their feet. Good foot herbs include plantain (*Plantago lanceolata*) and aloe vera (*Aloe barbadensis*).

⊚ **Soak athletic feet in bleach.** That's what they do in New England. Use a quarter cup of bleach for each quart of water, and soak your feet for twenty minutes once a day until your athlete's foot clears up.

⊚ **Spice up cold feet.** To warm up cold feet, North Carolina residents sometimes put pepper in their shoes. Sprinkle a small amount of cayenne (*Capsicum*

❧ Take a Garlic Foot Bath ❧

Seventh Day Adventists and other groups long have declared that garlic (*Allium sativum*) cures fungal infections. They're right, although how they figured it out is a mystery. Scientists have recently concluded that garlic's main antimicrobial constituent, allicin, can wipe out more than 40 types of bacteria, viruses, molds, fungi, and parasites. But allicin is released only when a garlic clove is cut, crushed, or otherwise broken apart.

To try this smelly cure, blend two garlic bulbs in a blender and add a quart of hot water. Fill a small tub with enough water to cover your feet. Add the hot garlic water, and soak for 20 minutes every evening until your condition disappears. Towel your feet briskly after each soak.

annuum) in your socks before going out in cold weather. Bring along a clean pair of socks in case the red pepper becomes irritating or painful.

⟳ **Warm them from the inside out.** Another foot-warming spice is cinnamon (*Cinnamomum zeylanicum*), which Chinese folk healers brew as a tea to prevent cold hands and feet. Stir one gram of powdered cinnamon in a glass of hot water and steep for fifteen minutes. Drink three times a day.

⟳ **Try some *huang qi*.** Huang qi, the Chinese name for astragalus root, is a mysterious herb that can make cattle loco if they eat too much of it. Nonetheless, it works wonders for cold human hands and feet. Astragalus (*Astragalus membranaceus*) roots are long and yellowish and look somewhat like popsicle sticks. Place three or four in one pint of water, bring to a boil, and simmer until one-third of the liquid disappears. Strain and drink two cups a day during cold weather.

Headache

The pain of a headache can be steady, piercing, or throbbing; its severity can range from minor discomfort to debilitation. Tension headaches and migraines are the most common types. Stress, irregular sleep, hormonal shifts, depression, eyestrain, and certain foods, among other things, can trigger a headache.

Conventional medicine usually combines medications with exercise and stress-reduction techniques to prevent and treat headaches.

Think away your pain. Yes, you can use your mind to heal your head. With biofeedback training, you can learn to control certain involuntary bodily functions, such as heart rate and body temperature, which can contribute to headaches. Take relaxation lessons from a biofeedback trainer and then practice at home. Wear loose clothing and sit in a comfortable chair. Close your eyes and imagine you are progressively tightening and then releasing all of your muscles, from your toes to the crown of your head.

Poke holes in it, the Chinese way. Acupuncture works well to cure headaches, especially chronic ones like migraines. By inserting needles at specific points on the body, the acupuncturist promises to restore the flow of *qi*, the vital life force, throughout the body. Now able to heal itself, the body weathers any stressors that might otherwise cause headaches.

Pinch yourself. Scared of needles? You can gain benefits similar to those offered through acupuncture by practicing a touch therapy known as acupressure. For a headache, squeeze the energy point known as L14, on the web between the thumb and index finger. You'll also find relief by massaging GB20, located on the back of the head at the base of the skull.

LEAF YOUR HEADACHE BEHIND

Say goodbye to migraine pain by chowing down on a feverfew sandwich. In the late 1970s, the wife of the chief medical officer of Great Britain's National Coal Board suffered greatly from migraine headaches. A local miner heard about her problem and told her that he'd also been a long-time migraine sufferer until he started chewing a couple of feverfew (*Tanacetum parthenium*) leaves each day. How the miner heard about this folk remedy is a mystery, but the woman tried it and noticed almost immediate relief. It's best to eat fresh leaves. Grow some in your garden. Then roll a few leaves up in a piece of bread and munch away to prevent or treat a migraine.

Get your neck straight. Even though it's your head that's hurting, a chiropractor is likely to relieve the pain by manipulating vertebrae in the neck.

Sit lotus-style. If you regularly practice the postures and breathing of yoga, you'll have fewer headaches, and the ones you get will be less severe.

Say hello to rosemary. Herbs containing rosmarinic acid act as anti-inflammatory agents, just like aspirin, ibuprofen, and acetaminophen do. These headache-busting herbs include rosemary

(*Rosmarinus officinalis*) and sage (*Salvia officinalis*).
Crush a handful of herbs and rub them on your temples
or head. Believe it or not, the remedy works. Or, if
you're reluctant to make a spectacle of yourself out in
the garden, brew up herbal teas or add the plants to
your bathwater.

Be a sourpuss. The Amish soak a cloth in full-
strength vinegar, wring it out, gently apply it to the
forehead, and lie down for 15 minutes to soothe headache pain.

Heart Disease

Coronary artery disease is a condition in which the
coronary arteries—the vessels that bring blood to
the heart muscle—become clogged with deposits of fat,
cholesterol, and other substances, collectively known as
plaque, which deprive the heart muscle of the blood it
needs. When the heart is in this weakened, malfunc-
tioning state, chest pain and a heart attack may result.
Early heart disease may have no symptoms. Warning
signs of a heart attack include severe chest pain, radiat-
ing to the neck, abdomen, or left arm; weakness; dizziness; sweating; nausea; and shortness of breath.
Conventional medicine treats heart conditions with
lifestyle changes, drug therapy, and surgery. It's important to keep in mind that, while the following healing
treatments can play a role in helping your heart, you

should not use them in place of traditional medical care prescribed by a physician.

Make a wish. What if you could heal yourself just by wishing it were so? Some heart patients have shown improvement after learning and practicing guided imagery and creative visualization in which they focused on images of clear arteries and a healthy heart.

Take traditional Chinese therapy to heart. Chinese physicians say heart disease may result from a deficiency of *yang* energy. To strengthen *yang*, they prescribe acupuncture, moxibustion, and herbs such as ginseng (*ren shen*) and aconite (*fu zi*). It's odd that aconite would help; it's a highly toxic herb (and therefore should only be administered by a qualified practitioner). Both acupuncture and acupressure can also help to lower blood cholesterol levels and ease other symptoms of heart disease.

Help yourself with Indian medicine. Yoga poses and breathing exercises are playing increasing roles in many heart programs around the country.

Take an orange break. Just sniffing an orange can lower blood pressure and anxiety and normalize an irregular heart beat. And aromatherapists say you don't even have to buy the essential oil. Simply peel an orange and inhale.

Add berries to your diet. Hawthorn (*Crataegus* spp.) berries appear to normalize heart function and eliminate chest pain by widening the arteries. Europeans have been using the berries for centuries.

Find help in nature. Eating a clove or two of garlic (*Allium sativum*) can lower your cholesterol levels and prevent blood clots from forming. Ginger also has cholesterol-lowering powers, and ginkgo (*Ginkgo biloba*) facilitates blood flow. (If you are on any medications for your heart, be sure to talk to your doctor before adding these to your diet.)

Run up your phone bill. That's not a pitch for your phone company. Recent research has actually shown that having a variety of social relationships

TAKING YOUR PULSE THE TIBETAN WAY

When you visit a Western doctor, he or she routinely takes your pulse to determine your heart rate. In Tibet, pulses along the ulnar artery in the forearm are taken to assess more esoteric conditions, such as involvement of spirits, health of relatives, and the patient's potential life span. The pulse is regarded as a messenger that tells the physician the condition of the body and its organs.

and regular contact with others can help protect you from a wide range of potentially fatal diseases. One study even found that people with lots of friends had significantly less blockage of their coronary arteries than did those individuals who reported having very little social support in their lives.

Hemorrhoids

Hemorrhoids are enlarged blood vessels under the lining of the rectum and anus. They are similar to varicose veins in that they are vessels that allow blood to pool. Hemorrhoids can result from extended periods of inactivity, straining to have bowel movements, chronic diarrhea, obesity, or pregnancy. Symptoms may include bleeding from the anus, pain and itching around the anus, or painful bowel movements. Conventional doctors recommend adding fiber to the diet, taking drugs to ease pain, or using soothing ointments to reduce tissue inflammation.

Add oil. Several essential oils, including cypress, geranium, and myrrh, will help hemorrhoids if used in compresses or sitz baths.

Swallow a little poison. A homeopath might give you minuscule doses of the poisons nux vomica and belladonna. Strangely, larger doses of these substances would cause hemorrhoids in a healthy person.

Seek aid from India. Some yoga exercises relieve constipation and improve circulation, which helps hemorrhoids to heal.

Cover them with carrots. You read it right. To treat hemorrhoids, New Englanders grate a small carrot and mix in enough lard to hold the shreds together in a sort of bolus, which is inserted in the anus and held in place as long as possible.

Treat them to a Russian steam bath. Eat onions to get rid of hemorrhoids, many people say. Seventh Day Adventists, for example, recommend eating cooked onions to stop bleeding. But along a much more unusual vein, Russian folklore calls for steaming hemorrhoids with fumes of cooked onions. Peel and chop four large onions and add to half a gallon of milk in a large pot. Cover and place in the oven on low heat. Remove the pot from the oven and remove the lid. Cover the pot with a toilet seat—if you have one handy—and sit down, or hover above the pot. Be very careful not to burn yourself on the steam or the pot. Complete the treatment by applying petroleum jelly to the hemorrhoids.

Pickle them. The Amish use alum to treat hemorrhoids. Alum is a sulphate of potassium and aluminum that occurs in crystalline form and is sometimes found in caves. It's used to make gunpowder, as a mordant to set dyes, and as an ingredient that makes pickles crisp. Just imagine what it does to your hemorrhoids. Fill a tub with enough water to cover your hips, as warm as you can stand. Add one cup of alum and stir thoroughly. Soak yourself for fifteen minutes. Dry off well.

Plant your bottom. Herbs good for treating hemorrhoids include witch hazel (*Hamamelis virginiana*), raspberry leaf (*Rubus idaeus*), mullein leaf (*Verbascum thapsus*), chamomile, (*Matricaria recutita*), yarrow (*Achillea millefolium*), horse chestnut (*Aesculus hippocastanum*), calendula (*Calendula officinalis*), and aloe vera. They are generally applied as a tea, gel, or salve directly to the hemorrhoids.

How to Make a Salve

Add hemorrhoid-healthy herbs to fat to make a soothing ointment. Salves are fat-based preparations used to soothe abrasions, heal wounds and lacerations, and soften dry, rough skin and chapped lips.

To make a hemorrhoid salve, chop, powder, crush, or grind herbs finely and place in a skillet or Crock-Pot with lard, butter, or another fat. If you're using a leafy herb, leave the mixture on the lowest heat for twenty minutes. If you're making a salve from roots, simmer for sixty minutes. Cool and refrigerate, using as needed.

Use beeswax instead of fat for a more permanent salve that you don't have to refrigerate.

High Blood Pressure

High blood pressure, or hypertension, describes a greater-than-normal force of blood coursing through the arteries. This higher pressure forces the heart to work harder than normal and increases the risk of aneurysm (rupture of an artery), heart attack, stroke, kidney failure, and other disorders. A reading of more than 140/90 is considered high. High blood pressure produces no symptoms in most people. Occasionally people with high blood pressure experience ringing in the ears or headaches. Conventional medical doctors attempt to lower blood pressure by prescribing drug therapy and lifestyle changes.

Let a Chinese doctor stick it to you. Sounds strange, but inserting hair-thin needles in specific points on your body, particularly in an area known as the "heart meridian," can lower blood pressure—for months or years.

Get a rubdown. It could help save your life. Massage works well to relieve stress, which can aggravate high blood pressure.

Raid the garden. Many common plants appear to have the power to lower or normalize blood pressure in some people. Garlic (*Allium sativum*) may bring down your blood pressure, reduce levels of harmful cholesterol, and "thin" your blood, which could prevent heart attacks. And if you spice up your life by eating more cayenne (*Capsicum annuum*), you may dilate your arteries and reduce blood pressure. Other helpful plants include hawthorn (*Crataegus* spp.) and ginkgo (*Ginkgo biloba*).

Put the squeeze on. It may not make sense to those of us used to conventional Western medicine, but acupressurists say that pressing on a point called Pericardium 2 can help to relax your body and lower your blood pressure to boot. The point is found in the elbow crease, directly above the ring finger. Pressing on Spleen 6—located four finger-widths above the inside of the anklebone—also may help to normalize blood pressure.

Sniff out a lower blood-pressure reading. Remarkably, just smelling certain scents can lower your blood pressure. Essential oils used to lower blood pressure include lavender (*Lavandula angustifolia*), rose (*Rosa* spp.), geranium (*Pelargonium graveoloens*), and sandalwood (*Santalum album*).

Get yourself a four-legged friend. Amazing as it sounds, simply caring for or petting a dog or cat has been shown to decrease blood pressure. So let that cat curl up on your lap or that puppy cuddle in your arms. Who would have dreamed that taking your medicine could be so safe—and enjoyable!

Impotence

Impotence is the inability of a man's penis to become erect or stay erect during sexual intercourse. In many cases, there's a psychological reason, including stress, depression, and relationship problems. Other causes include certain drugs, fatigue, a hormone imbalance, spinal-cord injury, or diabetes. Counseling is often effective if psychological factors are causing the problem. Otherwise, treatment includes drugs and/or surgery.

 Get your spine an adjustment. What's your spine got to do with how you perform in bed?

❧ HOW HOMEOPATHY CAN HELP ❧

Homeopathic medicine holds promise for men with impotence, particularly for cases stemming from anxiety and other psychological reasons. This strange therapy uses highly diluted doses of natural substances that would make a man impotent if given in full strength. The substances are derived from plant, animal, and mineral sources.

A homeopath also would try to pinpoint the cause of impotence by asking questions, such as, "Has there been a recent illness?" or "What are your feelings about sex and about your relationship?"

Chiropractors have helped many men to overcome impotence by manipulating the vertebrae in their spinal column.

Have it both ways. Some men have found relief from alternating hot and cold sitz baths or short soaks in ice-cold water.

Get your head in the game. Think your mind doesn't matter? It does. Biofeedback training, creative visualization, hypnotherapy, meditation, and other therapies bring body and mind together to relax a man and encourage successful and enjoyable intercourse.

Seek an ancient Chinese secret. Traditional Chinese medical treatment seeks to eliminate impotence by bringing qi, the body's energizing life force, back into balance. One possible explanation for impotence is that it results from a deficiency of yang, or male energy, in the kidney system. Together, yang and yin create harmony in the body. A typical Chinese physician would treat impotence with a combination of acupuncture, moxibustion, herbal therapy, and dietary changes.

Let plants perk you up. Saw palmetto (Serenoa repens) berries, from a small, unassuming palm tree native to the southeastern coast of the United States, have long been used as a remedy for enlarged prostate. Some men swear that the berries have aphrodisiacal powers as well. Ginseng (*Panax ginseng*) is used extensively throughout Asia and the United States to make a man feel young again. There is no scientific evidence that any plant can stimulate sexual desire. Nonetheless, many men say that such herbs have helped them to regain sexual prowess.

 Turn up the heat. Reach for the shaker of cayenne pepper on your spice rack and sprinkle the herb on a romantic dinner. Because of its hot character, cayenne has a reputation for getting the fires of passion burning.

Incontinence

Incontinence is the inability to control either urination, bowel movements, or both. There are several types of urinary incontinence. Causes range from infections and bladder stones to injury caused by childbirth or surgery. Bowel incontinence can result from a blockage of stool, severe diarrhea, or injury. Symptoms may include involuntary passing of urine; small pieces of stool or watery stool; and leaking urine after coughing, sneezing, lifting, or straining. Conventional treatment may consist of drug therapy, surgery, special exercises, and/or lifestyle changes.

 Put your mind in control. Who would have thought that you could use your head to treat incontinence? Biofeedback training can help people with incontinence to regain control over the muscles that regulate urination or bowel movements. The treatment uses monitors that "feed back" information on certain physical markers. Armed with this information, patients can learn to alter and control what once were considered to be involuntary body functions.

Weed the garden. Common weeds can help you to control incontinence. Plants known as "toning herbs" can strengthen and restore mucous membranes in the urinary tract, helping to correct or prevent incontinence. Particularly effective are the stems of horsetail (*Equisetum arvense*), taken in juice, as powder in capsules, or as an alcohol-based tincture. Other beneficial herbs include buchu (*Agathosma betulina*), corn silk (*Zea mays*), plantain (*Plantago lanceolata*), and nettle (*Urtica dioica*). Oddly enough, St. John's wort (*Hypericum perforatum*), a weed used by thousands of people to treat depression, is also added to herbal remedies for urinary incontinence. Many herbs may also be effective for treating ailments related to or precipitating incontinence, such as recurrent urinary-tract infections, constipation, and diarrhea; see an experienced herbalist for more on these.

Add some life force to your kidneys. Traditional Chinese physicians believe that incontinence is caused by a deficiency of *qi*, or life force, in the kidney. An acupuncturist will attempt to correct imbalances in the flow of *qi* by stimulating energy points on the body with hair-thin needles.

Give your kid something to chew on. Feeding a child watermelon or pumpkin seeds is said to cure bedwetting. Why? Who knows? But in rural areas the practice is said to be highly effective.

Memory Problems

Decreased blood flow to the brain can cause a variety of symptoms, including difficulties in concentration and memory, absentmindedness, confusion, lack of energy, fatigue, decrease in physical performance, depression, anxiety, dizziness, tinnitus (ringing in the ears), and headache. This collection of problems is known as cerebral insufficiency. Memory problems may also result from injury to the brain or from illnesses, such as Alzheimer's disease. Many people assume that they will experience memory problems as they grow older. But doctors tell us that memory problems do not necessarily go hand in hand with aging. If you take care of yourself, you have every reason to expect that your memory will be sharp and clear when you're ninety years old.

Remember rosemary. Rosemary (*Rosmarinus officinalis*) has a long history as an herb said to sharpen memory, concentration, and creativity, although there is no scientific data to back up the claim. In ancient times, brides even carried rosemary on their wedding day in the hope that their husbands would never forget them.

⊚ **Take advantage of an ancient Asian treasure.** The oldest tree on earth may help to boost your memory. Ginkgo (*Ginkgo biloba*) is a species that has thrived since dinosaurs roamed the planet. In China, Japan, and other Asian countries, ginkgo long has been prized as a memory booster. In the United States, the herb has enjoyed increasing popularity in recent years as Baby Boomers have sought to sharpen their memories. Scientists say ginkgo increases blood flow to the brain. Thus, it makes sense to take it for memory. Ginkgo also holds promise as a treatment for the debilitating Alzheimer's disease, which "erases" much of a person's memory and personality.

MEMORY FORMULA

To boost your memory and make it razor sharp, try this formula recommended by aromatherapists:

    10 drops rosemary oil
     6 drops lemon oil
     1 drop clary sage oil
     2 ounces distilled water

Combine all ingredients and use as an air spray.

⊚ **Let your nose remember for you.** Smells can trigger all sorts of physical responses, although scientists can't say why. To improve memory, aromatherapists suggest sniffing essential oils of sage (*Salvia officinalis*), clary sage (*Salvia sclarea*), basil (*Ocimum basilicum*), and bay laurel (*Laurus nobilis*). Trying to commit something to memory? Take a whiff of one of these scents as you repeat the information to yourself. Then, when you need to recall it, take a sniff of the same scent.

Mouth & Tooth Problems

Dental problems are among mankind's oldest afflictions. Anthropologists have discovered human skulls from 25,000 years ago that show signs of tooth decay. When it comes to dental problems, prevention is the best medicine. That means cleaning your teeth regularly and eating a healthy diet, with lots of fruits and vegetables. Unfortunately, our modern processed foods contain sugar and other chemicals that promote tooth decay. The primary risk of untreated dental decay is a dental abscess, an infection at the roots of the tooth in the jawbone. Such a condition can lead to systemic infection, causing health problems far beyond the site of the original infection. An abscess may require removal of the tooth, a root canal operation, and/or antibiotic therapy.

Cover it with clove. This common kitchen spice (*Syzgium aromaticum*) has been used as a tooth-pain remedy for thousands of years, particularly in Asia, where the tree originates. Today dentists use eugenol, the primary constituent of cloves, to treat dental pain. The chemical has natural anesthetic properties. The question is, how did ancient peoples know this? Cloves are still used in the folk medicine of New Englanders, Hispanics, and the Amish. Moisten one teaspoon powdered clove in olive oil and pack it into an aching dental cavity. Or purchase clove oil at any pharmacy, soak a cotton ball with it, and place the ball on the gums next to a bad tooth.

Accept a gift from the Magi. Another ancient dental remedy is myrrh, one of the gifts the Three Wise Men supposedly brought to the Christ child. Myrrh gum (*Commiphora myrrha*) has been used to treat mouth problems in the Middle East and North Africa since ancient times. Combine one and a half ounces myrrh gum and one teaspoon cayenne pepper (*Capsicuum annum*) with a pint of brandy. Cover the jar and shake several times a day for a week. Strain and use the liquid to treat toothache. Dip a cotton ball in the tincture and place it on or near a cavity. You can also use this herbal medicine to treat swollen and inflamed gums. Make a mouthwash by combining one ounce of the tincture with three ounces of water. Rinse your mouth with the wash frequently throughout the day.

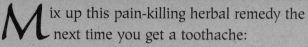

TOOTHACHE OIL

Mix up this pain-killing herbal remedy the next time you get a toothache:

    4 drops clove oil
    1 drop orange oil
    1 teaspoon vegetable oil

Combine all ingredients. Rub the oil onto painful gums. Repeat the treatment every half hour or so, as needed.

Chew on a tree. Chomping on other plants may help your dental problems, too. A number of trees and shrubs have been used to treat toothache, including willow (*Salix* spp.), goldenseal (*Hydrastis canadensis*), prickly ash (*Zanthoxylum americanum*), and yerba mansa (*Anemopsis californica*).

Look to the East to get rid of mouth odor. To banish bad breath, follow the Middle Eastern custom of chewing cardamom (*Elettaria cardamomum*) seeds.

Pour salt in your wound. New Englanders rinse their mouths with salt water to treat bleeding gums, canker sores, and toothache. You'll find the remedy in North Carolina as well. Dissolve one teaspoon of salt in a cup of warm water and rinse your mouth with it. North Carolinians sometimes place a teaspoon of salt directly on a sore tooth.

⊙ **Use a pack from the pantry.** Another unlikely remedy from North Carolina calls for packing a sore tooth with baking soda. It's a custom practiced in Hispanic communities in Los Angeles as well.

⊙ **Try a well-traveled remedy.** Sometimes folk medical customs have long and unusual origins. Mexicans and Hispanic-Americans in the United States sometimes cut a fig in half and lay it lengthwise between the cheek and an aching tooth. The remedy originated with Arabs, who took it to Spain. The Spaniards then brought it with them to the New World.

⊙ **Talk to the one who speaks.** Jewish-Americans suffering from toothaches have been known to seek help from an old woman known as a *Sprecherke* ("one who speaks"). The woman prays that the pain will be healed—and, miraculously, it often is.

Pain

Pain is a sign that your body has been harmed by disease, injury, or abnormal changes. Pain can range from mild irritation to excruciating agony. Pain is among the most commonly reported symptoms and is linked to innumerable disorders and diseases. It can be acute, such as after an injury, or chronic, as with arthritis. Conventional medicine primarily relies on drug therapy or surgery to relieve pain.

Counter the pain with cayenne. It's hard to believe that a substance that causes discomfort can help to relieve pain. Bite into a cayenne pepper (*Capsicum annuum*), and you'll imagine that your tongue is on fire. But apply cayenne externally, in a lotion, ointment, salve, or liniment, and it will help relieve many types of pain. The remedy is found in China and throughout the southwestern and midwestern United States.

Continue the herbal tradition. Many herbs have long been used to effectively relieve pain, although we may not know why. These include cramp bark (*Viburnum prunifolium*), willow bark (*Salix* spp.), ginger (*Zingiber officinalis*), rosemary (*Rosmarinus officinalis*), angelica (*Angelica archangelica*), and meadowsweet (*Filipendula ulmaria*).

Sample a South Pacific pain reliever. In the islands of the South Pacific, kava kava (*Piper methysticum*) is said to be a gift from the gods. The slightly narcotic herb is used in rituals to banish depression and lift the spirits. Oddly enough, kava kava also can help to ease muscle pain. Other muscle salves may be made from herbs such as comfrey (*Symphytum officinale*) and ginger (*Zingiber officinale*).

Breathe deeply. No one understands why, but smelling certain essential oils can help to ease muscle aches, spasms, and inflammation. Oils to try include ginger (*Zingiber officinale*), marjoram (*Origanum majorana*), peppermint (*Mentha piperita*), and thyme (*Thymus vulgaris*).

Try a hands-on approach. It's natural to rub a spot that we've just bumped or massage an over-worked muscle. But there may be more to it than simply instinct. Massage can help muscles to expel toxic chemicals. Many bodywork therapies can ease muscle pain and restore muscle function. Massage is particularly recommended to relieve muscle pain and tension.

Press the point. Reflexology, a type of massage, applies pressure to certain reflex points on the feet and hands to help the body heal itself. Shiatsu, a Japanese therapy, involves finger pressure at certain points on the body—often places nowhere near the site of discomfort—to ease pain and improve circulation.

Find relief with Chinese anesthesia. Traditional Chinese doctors say most traumatic injuries or painful conditions result from a stagnation of *qi*, the body's vital life force. *Qi* must flow freely through the body—even though nobody can see it. If *qi* becomes stagnant, then there is no movement, and pain results. To get *qi* moving again, Chinese doctors prescribe acupuncture stimulation. Acupuncture has been shown to help relieve pain. Indeed, in many Chinese hospitals, acupuncture has been used in place of anesthesia to relieve pain during and after surgery.

Flip a mental switch. There is no "switch" in our brains controlling painful sensations. But if you imagine that there is—and then mentally turn the switch off—you may attain some relief. Biofeedback training can be useful for muscle pain that refuses to go away, even after other conventional therapies have been tried. Biofeedback therapy teaches people to relax by tensing their muscles and then letting go. Patients also can learn to "switch off" pain signals in their brains. Guided-imagery and creative-visualization techniques are also effective in pain management and tension reduction.

Get entranced. Perhaps our minds are truly capable of helping us heal. Hypnosis, performed and taught by a professional medical hypnotherapist, has helped individuals suffering from chronic pain and addiction. The hypnotherapist may also teach you how to do self-hypnosis, so that you can take the pain relief with you.

Say Amen. Research has suggested that people who are recovering from surgery may heal more quickly or suffer fewer complications when they are being prayed for—even if they don't know the people saying the prayers and don't even know they're being prayed for. How could that be? No one knows for sure. But if you're dealing with pain from surgery or major injury, you may want to enlist the help of the faithful.

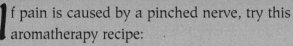

NERVE PAIN OIL

If pain is caused by a pinched nerve, try this aromatherapy recipe:

    4 drops chamomile oil
    5 drops marjoram oil
    5 drops helichrysum oil (optional)
    2 drops lavender oil
    1 ounce vegetable oil or St. John's wort oil

Combine all ingredients and store in a tightly capped jar. Apply as needed to relieve pain.

Look to England. In New England and parts of the Midwest, people sometimes take a bath with Epsom salt to relieve pain. The product is named after a salt found abundantly in spring water near the town of Epsom, England, in 1618. Epsom salt is reputed to have magical healing properties.

Butter up. Tibetan doctors mix butter with herbs such as cardamom (*Elettaria cardamomum*) and sandalwood (*Santalum album*) and apply the ointment to painful areas, such as the back. The herbs also may be powdered, burned, and inhaled to aid in healing pain.

Turn to a chiropractor. Many scientists are skeptical, but chiropractors say that adjusting misaligned spinal vertebrae can eliminate muscle pain and encourage the body to heal injured muscles.

Skin Conditions

Visible and uncomfortable, skin conditions demand attention. Perhaps that's why there are more traditional remedies for skin conditions than any other disorder. There are many types of skin problems, including acne, boils, dry skin, eczema, and itching and rashes, such as those caused by poison ivy and poison oak. Eczema is an inflammation of the skin characterized by red, oozing, sometimes crusty lesions on the face, scalp, and extremities. Conventional medicine uses drug therapy and/or lifestyle changes to treat many skin conditions.

Look to New England for relief from eczema. Seventh Day Adventists and New Englanders throw a few handfuls of baking soda in a warm bath and soak away their skin problems. The remedy is also used for relieving hives and other skin conditions.

Try a traditional Chinese poultice for acne. In China, folk healers treat acne by grinding dried mung beans, mixing the powder with water, and applying the poultice to the face, like a mask.

Reach for vinegar for poison ivy relief. Some people in Indiana and parts of Appalachia "wash away" poison ivy with vinegar. Vinegar, they say, works well to relieve any type of itching, including that caused by allergic rashes.

Pour coffee on yourself. No one has ever done scientific tests to determine why washing itchy skin with a strong cup of coffee has helped some people find relief from poison ivy.

Wash chapped hand with your breakfast. Next time your hands are chapped, try washing them with water and oatmeal instead of soap. After drying your hands with a towel, rub them again with dry oatmeal.

Use a Gypsy garlic cure. Gypsies use garlic paste as a treatment for all types of skin infections, impetigo, cuts, and other wounds. Pulverize three cloves of garlic (*Allium sativum*) in a blender or mortar. Add vinegar, a drop at a time, to make a thin paste. Apply to the infected area twice a day, leaving in place for fifteen minutes. Don't leave it on longer, or the paste may burn your skin. Wash the area thoroughly and cover with a clean dressing.

Smear on potato paste for puffiness. Gypsies have also been known to use potatoes to take puffiness out of skin. Potato poultices, they say, are particularly good for removing bags under the eyes. Clean and grate three unpeeled potatoes and press them with your hands to form a paste. Apply for fifteen minutes. Remove the paste and wash and dry the skin thoroughly.

WILD FIRE FLY!

Amish practitioners of Powwow medicine, a type of magic, employ a strange ritual to treat *Wildfeier* (wild fire), a red skin inflammation that doctors know as erysipelas.

Someone from the community, perhaps a neighbor child, is asked to represent the patient. The healer takes a red string, touches it to the top of the child's head, and brings it down over her body. The healer then sweeps the string from side to side three times, chanting:

"Wildfeier, flieh, flieh, flieh, Der Rode Fadem, jag dich hie, hie, hie!" (Wild fire, fly, fly, fly; the Red String chase you away, away, away!)

The Amish healer completes the ritual by burning the string.

Get milk. Milk relieves skin irritation and discomfort caused by a variety of ailments, say Hispanic-American folk healers in the Southwest. In the southern part of Appalachia, folks prefer buttermilk.

Rub a rind on baby's behind. If an Amish baby comes down with diaper rash, his mother might rub the infected area with a watermelon rind. She would then dry the baby's diaper area thoroughly and apply talcum powder.

Treat inflammation with an Incan tea. Inca healers used tea made from holly berries (*Ilex guayusa*, *Ilex paraguariensis*) to treat sunburn, reduce inflammation, and cleanse infected wounds.

Sleep Problems

Insomnia is the inability to get a good night's sleep. The condition has more to do with quality of sleep than quantity; in fact, some people need as little as four hours per night. Causes of insomnia may include mental anguish, breathing problems, uncomfortable or erratic sleeping arrangements, drug and alcohol misuse, digestive disorders, or depression. Conventional medicine's treatment program for insomnia depends on its causes. Drug therapy, psychotherapy, and/or lifestyle adjustments may be recommended.

Douse the "fire in your heart." Acupuncturists view insomnia as an imbalance of *qi*, the body's vital energy force. One possible explanation for insomnia is that it results from a deficiency of *yin* energy in the kidney system, causing "fire" in the heart system. Acupuncture aims to correct *qi* imbalances by stimulating energy flow with thin needles inserted in specific points on the body.

Squeeze your wrist. Acupressure operates along the same theories of vital energy as acupuncture.

The difference is that you can practice acupressure yourself at home. To get a good night's sleep, press a spot called Heat 7 on the inner arms along the wrist crease, in the hollow that is in line with the little fingers. Pericardium 6 is also on the inner arms, between the tendons, three finger-widths above the wrist crease. Press or massage in a small circle with your finger for thirty to sixty seconds.

Give yourself a Japanese thumb rub. A Japanese form of acupressure, known as jin shin jyutsu, calls for massaging the thumb gently until you relax and fall asleep.

Give valerian a try. For centuries, folk healers in Europe have prescribed the herb valerian (*Valeriana officinalis*) for sleeplessness. Studies show that valerian calms some people as effectively as the prescription drug Valium. The strange part is that some people who take the calming herb actually become agitated. No one knows why.

Pick a dilly remedy. A Chinese folk healer might wash your head in a tea made from dill seeds (*Anethum graveolens*). That way you can't help but smell the fumes, which are said to promote sleep. You will also end up smelling like a pickle. If that prospect is unappealing, try adding eight to ten drops of dill oil to one ounce of vegetable oil. Apply the mixture to a cloth and keep it near your nose when you go to bed.

● **Borrow your kitty's catnip.** Catnip (*Nepeta cataria*), a common weed that makes felines go bonkers, helps some people to fall asleep. American Indians drank catnip tea to drop off to sleep. The remedy is popular among Seventh Day Adventists, too.

● **Take a homeopathic coffee cure.** Homeopaths give insomniacs diluted substances that would cause insomnia in full strength, such as *coffea cruda*.

● **Tap into your brain.** Biofeedback training, relaxation therapy, and hypnosis can reduce anxiety and make it easier for you to get to sleep. It's mind over matter—and science can't tell you why it works.

● **Listen to Mother Nature.** Some people benefit from sound therapy, which uses natural sounds, such as waves on a beach or wind rustling leaves, to ease tension and anxiety before bedtime. Why do nature sounds soothe us? It's a mystery.

● **Sleep with an Old World cure.** Stuffing a pillow with soothing herbs is an old European remedy for sleeplessness. As herbal medicine has regained popularity in recent years, many people in the United States use herb pillows today. Children should sleep on pillows filled with mild herbs, such as lavender (*Lavandula angustifolia*), lemon balm (*Melissa officinalis*), chamomile (*Matricaria recutita*), and dill (*Anethum graveolens*). Adults may prefer pillows stuffed with hop

(*Humulus lupulus*), the herb that gives beer its bitter flavor.

⊚ **Temper your wind.** In Tibet, a patient with a "wind imbalance" that results in restlessness, sleeplessness, and frequent yawning might be advised to seek out a warm place and spend time with friends.

Sore Throat

A sore throat is a raw sensation in the back of the throat that makes swallowing painful. It may be a symptom of pharyngitis (inflammation of the throat) or streptococcal infection (strep throat). Often a sore throat is the first symptom of a cold, the flu, laryngitis (inflammation of the voice box), or another condition. A sore throat may also result from overuse (such as screaming) or abuse (smoking). In some instances, a sore throat may be caused by problems in the sinuses, lungs, or digestive tract. To stop the pain of a common sore throat, conventional doctors suggest taking aspirin, acetaminophen, or a nonsteroidal anti-inflammatory drug, such as ibuprofen. People with strep or bacterial infections need antibiotics, such as penicillin.

⊚ **Dress your throat like a lumberjack.** Mix two cups of hot water with two drops of lavender (*Lavandula angustifolia*) oil, two drops of bergamot (*Citrus bergamia*) oil, and one drop of tea tree

(*Melaleuca alternifolia*) oil. Soak a cloth—flannel works best—in the liquid, wring it out, and wrap the cloth around your sore throat.

Suck on some bark. *Ouch!* you say? Well, the bark from the slippery elm tree (*Ulmus fulva*) was used by American Indians and colonists as a remedy for sore throat. When moistened with water, slippery elm powder turns into a slimy goo that soothes the throat.

Take a tip from North Carolinians. Onion syrup is a popular remedy in New England and North Carolina. New Englanders cover sliced raw onions with sugar. The sugar draws out the moisture in the onions and forms a syrup. But this process can take a day or two. North Carolinians speed it up by placing the onion-sugar mixture in a baking pan and leaving it in the oven on low heat until the syrup forms. Either way, take one tablespoon, as needed.

Sample a well-traveled remedy. Indiana farmers have been known to suck a lemon sprinkled with salt. Surprisingly, Gypsies in Europe do the same thing, but they mix lemon juice with water-diluted salt.

Listen to the singers. For centuries, singers from European countries have gargled with marjoram (*Origanum majorana*) tea sweetened with honey.

◉ **Get steamed.** Aromatherapists might advise you to inhale steam from essential oils of sage (*Salvia officinalis*), hyssop (*Hyssopus officinalis*), thyme (*Thymus vulgaris*), lavender (*Lavandula angustifolia*), or eucalyptus (*Eucalyptus globulus*). Add a few drops of one or more oils to a bowl of hot water. Lean over the bowl with a towel draped over your head and breathe deeply.

Wounds & Cuts

When it comes to wounds and cuts, the goal is to stop the bleeding, clean the wound, and manage any resulting infection. Even the smallest scratch or can become infected. Superficial infections then can penetrate deeper into the body to form an abscess, which may spread into the bloodstream and harm internal organs. Besides cleaning a wound, a conventional doctor might also prescribe antibiotics or other drugs. (If you have diabetes or circulation problems, do not attempt to treat wounds yourself; see your doctor.)

◉ **Make it stink.** From ancient times, healers have washed wounds in garlic. It may not smell great, but it works, they say. First, clean the wound with soap and water. Next, using a blender, mix three garlic (*Allium sativum*) cloves with one cup of wine. Allow the mixture to stand for three hours, then strain. Apply the garlic preparation with a clean cloth. Cover with sterile gauze and tape. Repeat this process twice a day.

Brown bag it. Amish healers cut a piece from a brown paper bag and soak it in vinegar, then they apply it to the wound and cover it with a clean cloth.

Give yourself flowers. Aromatherapists recommend essential oil of lavender (*Lavandula angustifolia*) for treating wounds. Clean the wound thoroughly and apply the oil in a compress.

Use the other white meat. Less appealing is this remedy that dates to ancient Egypt and is still used by people in New England and the Midwest and by African-Americans in Louisiana. Wrap your wound in a piece of salt pork or fatback.

Raid your window box. An old European remedy for wounds is to wash them with a tea made from pot marigolds (*Calendula officinalis*). Fill a one-pint jar with boiling water and one ounce of marigold flowers. Cover tightly and steep until the liquid cools to room temperature. Strain and apply the tea to the wound with a clean cloth. Allow the wound to dry. Then cover it with sterile gauze. Do this several times a day, until the wound heals.

Start a fire. Seventh Day Adventists pulverize charcoal from a wood fire and apply it to wounds that are oozing pus. The poultice is covered with a bandage; the dressing should be changed every day.

INDEX